The Ankylosing Spondylitis Mastery Bible: Your Blueprint For Complete Ankylosing Spondylitis Management

Dr. Ankita Kashyap and Prof. Krishna N. Sharma

Published by Virtued Press, 2023.

While every precaution has been taken in the preparation of this book, the publisher assumes no responsibility for errors or omissions, or for damages resulting from the use of the information contained herein.

THE ANKYLOSING SPONDYLITIS MASTERY BIBLE: YOUR BLUEPRINT FOR COMPLETE ANKYLOSING SPONDYLITIS MANAGEMENT

First edition. November 27, 2023.

Copyright © 2023 Dr. Ankita Kashyap and Prof. Krishna N. Sharma.

ISBN: 979-8223334064

Written by Dr. Ankita Kashyap and Prof. Krishna N. Sharma.

Table of Contents

- 1
- Introduction 2
- Understanding Ankylosing Spondylitis 4
- What Is Ankylosing Spondylitis? 5
- The Pathophysiology of Ankylosing Spondylitis 8
- Early Signs and Symptoms 11
- Diagnostic Procedures 13
- Impact on the Spine and Joints 17
- Psychological and Emotional Effects 20
- Quality of Life Implications 22
- Medical Management of Ankylosing Spondylitis 24
- Non-Steroidal Anti-Inflammatory Drugs (NSAIDs) 25
- Disease-Modifying Antirheumatic Drugs (DMARDs) 27
- Biological Therapies 30
- Physical Therapy and Rehabilitation 33
- Exercise and Stretching 36
- Surgical Interventions 38
- Complementary and Alternative Medicine 41
- Holistic Approaches to Ankylosing Spondylitis Management 45
- The Role of Nutrition in Ankylosing Spondylitis 46
- Exercise and Movement Therapy 49
- Stress Management and Relaxation Techniques 52
- Sleep Optimization 54
- Heat and Cold Therapies 57
- Mind-Body Techniques 59
- Supportive Therapies 63
- Creating a Personalized Ankylosing Spondylitis Management Plan 66
  - Assessing Your Symptoms and Needs 67
  - Setting Realistic Goals 70
  - Building a Support Network 73

Developing Self-Care Techniques 76
Adapting to Flare-Ups 79
Monitoring and Tracking Progress 81
Adjusting the Management Plan 84

DISCLAIMER

The information provided in this book is intended for general informational purposes only. The content is not meant to substitute professional medical advice, diagnosis, or treatment. Always consult with a qualified healthcare provider before making any changes to your management plan or healthcare regimen.

While every effort has been made to ensure the accuracy and completeness of the information presented, the author and publisher do not assume any responsibility for errors, omissions, or potential misinterpretations of the content. Individual responses to management strategies may vary, and what works for one person might not be suitable for another.

The book does not endorse any specific medical treatments, products, or services. Readers are encouraged to seek guidance from their healthcare providers to determine the most appropriate approaches for their unique medical conditions and needs.

Any external links or resources provided in the book are for convenience and informational purposes only. The author and publisher do not have control over the content or availability of these external sources and do not endorse or guarantee the accuracy of such information.

Readers are advised to exercise caution and use their judgment when applying the information provided in this book to their own situations. The author and publisher disclaim any liability for any direct, indirect, consequential, or other damages arising from the use of this book and its content.

By reading and using this book, readers acknowledge and accept the limitations and inherent risks associated with implementing the strategies, recommendations, and information contained herein. It is always recommended to consult a qualified healthcare professional for personalized medical advice and care.

Introduction

Title: The Ultimate Guide to Ankylosing Spondylitis: Your Comprehensive Guide to Ankylosing Spondylitis Management —-

Greetings, Reader

Do you ever find yourself longing for an end to the constant pain that appears to be consuming every part of your being? Have you ever pondered if there's a way to reclaim control over your body, your life, and your future as you stared into the mirror, your eyes bearing the weight of this chronic condition?

I still recall my initial interaction with a patient who was struggling with the effects of ankylosing spondylitis. On this muggy July afternoon, there was a strong stench of doubt in the air. Their eyes, which showed a complex mixture of fear, resignation, and a glimmer of hope, revealed this tough person sitting across from me. I became aware of the seriousness of the adventure we were going to take together at that very moment.

Ankylosing Spondylitis is a persistent nemesis that lurks in the background and is frequently misdiagnosed and disregarded. It's a disorder that defies explanation, necessitating a comprehensive strategy that goes beyond normal medical practise. The myths and difficulties surrounding its administration are as varied as the people who must carry its burden. A route that leads to empowerment and control over this affliction is beckoned to be embraced by a beacon of hope within this complex tapestry of problems.

When faced with the difficult task of controlling Ankylosing Spondylitis, the majority of people frequently take a well-traveled route that results in temporary fixes. I've seen innumerable people struggle to overcome the constraints of traditional management as they make their way through a labyrinth of general recommendations and insufficient strategies. Their frustration is evident. I am thinking of one patient in particular, Lily. She had given in to the idea that her illness was an inflexible force and accepted that her life will be determined by its whims. But when Lily adopted a fresh viewpoint, her narrative took an incredible turn, one I can't wait to tell you about.

The true cure for Ankylosing Spondylitis is not found in the confines of traditional knowledge. It is found in the smooth fusion of medical knowledge with holistic health, a method that goes beyond the surface to the very centre of this illness. It's a journey that asks you to let go of the limitations of survival and embrace a vibrant, purpose-driven life.

I want you to imagine the possibilities that lie within the pages of this book as you hold it in your hands. This book is more than just a book; it's a friend and a lighthouse that shows you how to take back your life from Ankylosing Spondylitis. It is evidence of your fortitude and a steadfast pledge of assistance as you make your way through this condition's maze.

Let me describe it to you: Imagine yourself awakening one morning with a renewed sense of energy coursing through your body. The uneasy murmurs that used to fill every conscious second of your life have been replaced by a calm that seeps into your very being. It's a profoundly realising moment, proof of the insights discovered within these pages having the ability to transform.

The voyage we are about to take together will be nothing short of remarkable, I assure you, dear reader. You will experience a gradual unravelling of your personal storey with every page flip, creating a tapestry that speaks of resiliency, self-determination, and unshakable optimism.

Thus, let's go out on this journey together, as these pages include the instructions needed to conquer Ankylosing Spondylitis. The road ahead is full of opportunities, and I can't wait to travel with you as we reveal the mysteries that will mould your path to total control and unrestricted empowerment.

Regards for your well-being,
Dr. Ankita Kashyap

Understanding Ankylosing Spondylitis

What Is Ankylosing Spondylitis?

Welcome to the fascinating voyage of deciphering the riddles behind ankylosing spondylitis, dear reader. It is essential that we familiarise ourselves with the essential phrases that will lead us through the complex web of this condition before we set out on our exploration. Gaining an understanding of these terminologies will improve our understanding and facilitate a deeper understanding of the essence of Ankylosing Spondylitis.

To start, let us clarify some basic words that will serve as our compass on this exciting journey.

Spondylitis Ankylosing: This mysterious phrase refers to a long-term inflammatory illness that mostly affects the spine, resulting in pain, stiffness, and in extreme situations, the fusion of spinal vertebrae. Ankylosing Spondylitis affects not only the spine but also other joints and, in rare cases, important organs. It's a condition that requires consideration, sympathy, and comprehension.

Understanding prevalence and risk factors is essential to understanding the severity and range of ankylosing spondylitis. Prevalence is the frequency with which a given condition occurs in a given community, whereas risk factors are those that increase the chance of having a condition. We can appreciate the importance of Ankylosing Spondylitis and the possible paths toward proactive therapy and prevention when we are aware of its prevalence and risk factors.

Let us now explore the meanings of each of these terms separately and how they apply to Ankylosing Spondylitis.

Ankylosing Spondylitis: Visualize the spine as the stout trunk of a stately tree, giving the whole thing balance and elegance. Imagine now that this trunk is under attack from inflammation, becoming rigid and losing its suppleness. This captures the essence of ankylosing spondylitis, in which the spine acts as a battlefield for unrelenting inflammation, causing discomfort, limiting movement, and a significant impact on day-to-day functioning. Although it mostly affects the spine, this disorder can also affect other joints, including the hips, shoulders, and knees, which can present a variety of difficulties for those who are affected.

Risk variables and prevalence: Understanding the prevalence of ankylosing spondylitis and the risk factors that go along with it becomes crucial as we navigate the terrain of the condition. Ankylosing spondylitis is not as common in all populations, however it is more common in some areas and among particular ethnic groups. Understanding the prevalence helps us understand the extent of the problem and the necessity for specialised treatment methods.

Furthermore, examining risk factors reveals a mosaic of elements that lead to the development of Ankylosing Spondylitis. The complex storey of this illness is shaped by a combination of immunological complexities, environmental variables, and genetic predisposition. Through the identification and comprehension of these risk factors, we may steer towards preventative measures that are proactive and individualised care plans.

Let's now weave a thread that ties these terms to well-known ideas and grounds them in relatability.

Imagine a symphony of movement, with the spine harmonising with the beat of daily life, if you have ankylosing spondylitis. Imagine now that discord is seeping into this symphony, forcing the spine to march to the rhythm of stiffness and inflammation. This captures the spirit of Ankylosing Spondylitis, in which life's music is tinted with discomfort and movement's orchestra is upset. We close the gap between the clinical language and the visceral sensations of patients living with Ankylosing Spondylitis by connecting the complexity of this ailment to the universal language of harmony and discord.

Risk variables and prevalence: Imagine a large mosaic in which every tile stands for a distinct aspect of the human experience. Now see the prevalence of Ankylosing Spondylitis as a patchwork inside this mosaic, depicting its effects on various populations in a variety of ways. The risk factors show the complex interactions between heredity, environment, and immune responses, and they are like the threads that weave through this mosaic, shaping the onset of Ankylosing Spondylitis. We give these concepts a sense of familiarity and resonance by entwining them with the imagery of a colourful mosaic, which helps to establish a closer bond with their core.

Let's pause as we weave our way through the storey of ankylosing spondylitis to consider this thought-provoking question:

How can we, as compassionate and understanding people, embrace the complexity of Ankylosing Spondylitis and create a supportive and empowering environment for individuals who must navigate its tortuous course?

This query acts as a lighthouse, pointing the way forward and encouraging us to learn more about the subtleties of ankylosing spondylitis. Come along with me as we peel back the layers of this fascinating journey in search of knowledge and understanding that will reveal the blueprint for managing Ankylosing Spondylitis from start to finish.

The Pathophysiology of Ankylosing Spondylitis

Let's peel back the years and explore the intriguing progression of this mysterious illness as we set off on our adventure into the complex world of Ankylosing Spondylitis. Resilience, mystery, and resilience are all interwoven in the pathophysiology of Ankylosing Spondylitis, from the disease's first historical whispers to its contemporary interpretations and adaptations.

Imagine being on the cusp of time, seeing the onset of a condition that will impact millions of lives. With its origins steeped in medical history, Ankylosing Spondylitis has long piqued the interest of medical professionals, academics, and seekers of knowledge.

Whispers of agony and stiffness in the spine reverberated through the halls of ancient civilizations, marking the oldest known beginnings of Ankylosing Spondylitis. References to a disease that resembles Ankylosing Spondylitis can be discovered in the whispers of medical scrolls and historical books, suggesting that this mysterious illness has a long history.

Time travel to the 17th century, when the great physician Bernard Connor first described the clinical characteristics of ankylosing spondylitis through his careful observations. Deeper comprehension of this illness is made possible by his unwavering drive to solving the mysteries of human physiology and his acute eye.

A new era of understanding was brought about in the 20th century with the identification of the HLA-B27 gene, a genetic marker that is strongly linked to Ankylosing Spondylitis. This significant achievement clarified the condition's genetic foundations and the complex dance between nature and nurture that contributes to its development.

Let us examine the complex human body as a starting point for our understanding search. Here, the interaction of genes, immune cells, and inflammatory mediators creates a clear picture of the pathophysiology of ankylosing spondylitis. Stars that point the way on this cosmic exploration tour include illustrations of the inflammatory cascade and the spine's role.

Traveling the world exposes us to the finer points and variances in the appearance of Ankylosing Spondylitis. The appearance and management of this illness are shaped by cultural and regional factors, creating a colourful and diverse mosaic. The diversity of human experiences is reflected in the cultural mosaic of Ankylosing Spondylitis, ranging from the holistic approaches of indigenous societies to the age-old therapeutic practises of the Far East.

The hidden landscapes of Ankylosing Spondylitis have been revealed in the modern period thanks to advancements in imaging technology, providing a glimpse into the complex network of inflammation and structural changes within the spine. Computed tomography (CT) scans and magnetic resonance imaging (MRI) have become indispensable instruments that let us see behind the curtain and observe the silent dance of sickness inside the body.

The care of Ankylosing Spondylitis has entered a new era with the introduction of biologic medicines, which take a targeted approach to modifying the immune response. These cutting-edge therapies revitalise worn-out joints and bones and provide a glimmer of hope to individuals navigating the intricate paths of persistent inflammation.

In the middle of the victories and triumphant arcs of development, we also need to recognise the difficulties and disagreements that dot the history of ankylosing spondylitis. The pursuit of prompt diagnosis and intervention persists as a compelling urge, drawing us to cross the divide between the onset of symptoms and the clarity of the diagnosis. The usage of non-steroidal anti-inflammatory medicines (NSAIDs) and its long-term effects on cardiovascular health have generated controversy, which highlights the need for a complete and nuanced approach to treating this problem.

We are urged to embrace the complexities and subtleties of ankylosing spondylitis as we stand on the brink of understanding and to create a compassionate and wise tapestry in our quest for holistic wellbeing and comprehensive management.

We will travel through the clinical signs and diagnostic processes of ankylosing spondylitis in the upcoming chapter, exploring the intricate paths of this illness and providing guidance for individuals who want to take control of their health and well-being.

Early Signs and Symptoms

As we dig into the complex tapestry of Ankylosing Spondylitis, welcome, my reader, to a journey of understanding and empowerment. Let us set out to decipher the mysterious symptoms and indicators that frequently go undetected in the initial phases, as the secret to preventive care is found in these faint indications from the body.

Picture a world in which a small town is bathed in a soft morning glow and the pulse of life pulses with a serene elegance. Our storey, which is one of resiliency and the pursuit of healing, takes place against this tranquil backdrop.

Introducing Sarah, a bright young lady whose dreams are as endless as the sky. Her laughter reverberates throughout her life, and her soul is limitless. However, she is unaware of it and neither is everyone around her of the silent battle that is brewing within her.

Sarah was unaware that the initial symptoms of Ankylosing Spondylitis had already started to delicately weave themselves throughout her body. Because this illness is so subtle, it frequently goes unnoticed, appearing as occasional soreness or light exhaustion. The main obstacle is to identify the faint signs of Ankylosing Spondylitis amid the noise of everyday existence, which can be found in these elusive murmurs.

Our strategy must be one of unwavering vigilance and gentle understanding in the pursuit of early diagnosis and intervention. We provide the groundwork for a proactive approach to combat the subtle progression of Ankylosing Spondylitis by combining medical knowledge with holistic well-being. Early intervention and empowered management are made possible by our combination of a thorough assessment of symptoms, customised lifestyle modifications, and individualised treatment.

Sarah has a fresh clarity as the caring wisdom of her healthcare team guides her as the tendrils of awareness unfold within her consciousness.

Sarah gains control over her well-being and a sense of empowerment through early detection and a comprehensive approach to management. Her spirit is nourished and a road to a resilient and hopeful future is laid by the tactful acceptance of proactive assistance.

The management storey of ankylosing spondylitis is reflected in Sarah's experience, which weaves a complex picture. The case study highlights the power of proactive management, the effectiveness of a comprehensive strategy, and the transforming effect of early identification. The statement invites contemplation regarding the importance of identifying the minute details of our physique and the far-reaching consequences of prompt intervention.

Ankylosing Spondylitis's sophisticated dance of early symptoms and indicators is a reflection of the complex relationship between proactive wellness and awareness. It calls us to learn how to listen to our bodies' subtle cues and to develop a harmonious body-mind-spirit synergy. The importance of early detection is woven into the larger storey of managing Ankylosing Spondylitis completely, creating a resilient and empowered fabric.

While we bask in the soft embrace of Sarah's journey, let us consider the enormous consequences of early identification and proactive care. In the world of inflammatory bowel disease, how may awareness of subtle symptoms and indicators fan the flame of empowerment? Inspired by the subtle hints of empowerment and understanding, we set out on a mission to piece together the mysterious fabric of early detection and proactive wellbeing.

In the sections that follow, we will skillfully and gracefully negotiate the maze of ankylosing spondylitis, creating a road map for total control over this mysterious illness. Let's go on this voyage.

Diagnostic Procedures

As we dig into the complex tapestry of Ankylosing Spondylitis, welcome, my reader, to a journey of empowerment and understanding. Let's set out to decipher the mysterious symptoms and indicators that frequently go undetected in the early phases because the secret to proactive management can be found in these subliminal cues from the body.

Imagine a place where a small village is bathed in a soft morning glow and where people go about their daily lives with a serene ease. Our story—one of resiliency and the pursuit of wellness—takes place against this tranquil backdrop.

Introducing Sarah, a vibrant young lady with aspirations as big as the sky. Her spirit has no boundaries, and her laughter reverberates throughout her life. However, she and all around her are unaware of the silent battle that is brewing inside her.

Sarah had no idea that the early symptoms of Ankylosing Spondylitis had started to tangle themselves delicately throughout her body. This illness is subtle and can appear as minor weariness or temporary discomfort. The main difficulty is to identify the faint signs of Ankylosing Spondylitis amid the noise of everyday existence, which can be found in these elusive murmurs.

Our approach must be one of unwavering vigilance and gentle understanding in the goal of early diagnosis and intervention. By merging medical knowledge with holistic health, we provide the groundwork for a proactive approach to combating Ankylosing Spondylitis's sneaky progress. We create the conditions for early intervention and self-managed care by combining a thorough assessment of symptoms, customised lifestyle changes, and individualised care.

A newfound clarity appears as the caring knowledge of Sarah's healthcare team guides the tendrils of awareness to unfold within her consciousness. Sarah feels empowered and has agency over her health because to early detection and a comprehensive care strategy. Her soul is nourished by the kind embrace of proactive intervention, which also clears the way for a resilient and hopeful future.

The larger storey of managing ankylosing spondylitis is reflected in the fabric of Sarah's experience. The case study highlights the importance of early discovery, the effectiveness of a comprehensive strategy, and the game-changing potential of proactive management. It challenges us to consider the importance of appreciating the minute details of our bodies and the far-reaching effects of early action.

The complicated relationship between proactive wellbeing and awareness is reflected in the delicate dance of early indications and symptoms within the realm of Ankylosing Spondylitis. It invites us to develop a harmonic synergy between mind, body, and spirit by learning to embrace the art of listening to the whispers of our bodies. The importance of early detection is woven into the larger storey of managing Ankylosing Spondylitis completely, creating a resilient and empowered whole.

Let us consider the significant ramifications of early detection and effective management as we linger in the comforting embrace of Sarah's journey. In the world of Ankylosing Spondylitis, how may the awareness of subtle signs and symptoms fan the flame of empowerment? Inspired by these words, we set out on a mission to decipher the mysterious fabric of proactive wellbeing and early detection, led by the soft murmurs of empowerment and comprehension.

Within these pages, we will gracefully and tenaciously navigate the maze of Ankylosing Spondylitis, creating a road map for total control over this mysterious illness. Now let's start our journey.

1. : The first step in the diagnostic process is a detailed physical examination conducted by a healthcare professional. This may entail determining your range of motion, examining the locations of your pain and inflammation, and looking for any indications of stiffness or discomfort in your spine. Your healthcare professional will obtain

important information via careful palpation and observation, which will guide the next diagnostic procedures.

2.: To see the structural alterations in the spine and sacroiliac joints, imaging tests including X-rays, CT (Computerized Tomography) scans, and MRIs are frequently used after the physical examination. By taking a deeper look at the skeletal structures, these non-invasive methods can identify any distinctive patterns linked to Ankylosing Spondylitis.

3.: A number of blood tests are essential to the diagnosis procedure, including as the HLA-B27 test and markers of inflammation such erythrocyte sedimentation rate (ESR) and C-reactive protein (CRP). These tests help confirm the diagnosis of Ankylosing Spondylitis by providing important information regarding the existence of inflammation and immune system activation.

- Embrace the process: Diagnosing someone else can be a scary and difficult process. You can approach the process with resilience and courage if you embrace each phase with an open mind and heart.

- Communicate openly: It's critical to have open lines of communication with your healthcare staff. Discuss any worries, symptoms, or inquiries you may have; doing so will encourage a cooperative and encouraging attitude to your treatment.

When the diagnostic processes are successfully completed, you and your healthcare team will have a thorough understanding of your situation. The combination of the results of your blood tests, imaging studies, and physical examination will confirm that you have ankylosing spondylitis and direct your course of treatment.

It's critical to maintain patience and persistence throughout the diagnostic process in the event of unclear or inconclusive results. Your medical team will put forth great effort to investigate other options and deal with any obstacles that could come up.

We are getting a better picture of your health and well-being with every step we take as we make our way across the complex terrain of diagnostic procedures. Accept the process with poise and fortitude, knowing that each puzzle piece that is solved will point the way toward efficient administration and all-encompassing care.

Impact on the Spine and Joints

Imagine a calm morning when the world is still shrouded in the silence of dawn. Dappled patterns are created on the ground when the soft sunshine permeates through the leaves. This peaceful sight is surrounded by a quiet fight that is frequently ignored. This peaceful scene might be clouded by the pain, stiffness, and limited mobility that accompany Ankylosing Spondylitis, a disease that affects the spine and joints.

Join the main characters in this complex dance of perseverance and difficulty. The joints—those complex hinges that permit elegant movement—play an essential supporting role to the spine, which is the main structural element. The spine is a pillar of stability and flexibility. These essential elements serve as the setting for the storey of living with Ankylosing Spondylitis, a disease that can push a person's physical and mental boundaries.

The main obstacle is the subtle way that Ankylosing Spondylitis spreads through the spine and joints, causing pain and restriction. An ongoing companion, pain disrupts the peace of daily existence. Strictness envelops the body and limits mobility, akin to misty tendrils. Mobility turns as a valuable resource that frequently eludes grasp like sand grains.

A diverse strategy is necessary to meet these issues. This calls for a careful balancing act between lifestyle changes, medical interventions, and an all-encompassing approach to well-being. The cornerstones of this strategy are the use of targeted drugs to control inflammation, physical therapy to preserve strength and flexibility, and the addition of mild exercises to increase mobility. In addition, developing self-care practises and creating a supportive atmosphere can be quite helpful in overcoming the challenges presented by Ankylosing Spondylitis.

The outcomes of this strategy start to show as the individual threads come together, much like flowers do in a garden. Pain is reduced, allowing for brief intervals of comfort and relief. The grip of stiffness progressively relaxes, enabling more flexibility and range of motion.

Mobility, which was formerly only a pipe dream, starts to materialise and gives people back their sense of bodily freedom.

After some thought, it's evident that managing ankylosing spondylitis is not without its difficulties. Resilience and adaptation are necessary because the route is frequently paved with uncertainty and failures. However, the seeds of development and transformation are sowed right amid these difficulties. The knowledge gained along this journey is priceless, providing insights into the human spirit's resiliency and the effectiveness of a holistic approach to wellbeing.

Anatomical diagrams and pictures can be very helpful in providing insight into how Ankylosing Spondylitis affects the spine and joints. These tools can provide clarity and insight by graphically representing the changes in the body, which can improve the reader's comprehension of the condition and how to manage it.

The effects on the spine and joints are a microcosm of the larger storey of optimism and perseverance in the therapy of Ankylosing Spondylitis. It emphasises how crucial it is to take a holistic approach that takes into account a person's emotional and psychological health in addition to the condition's outward symptoms. A more holistic view of health and wellness is made possible by recognising the connection between the body and mind.

We are faced with an interesting conundrum as we learn more about the complex interactions between Ankylosing Spondylitis and the body: How can we keep encouraging resilience and a sense of empowerment in the face of such difficulties? This inquiry acts as a lighthouse, pointing the way for additional research and interaction with the deeply intricate details of Ankylosing Spondylitis and its treatment.

The effects on the spine and joints are a microcosm of the larger storey of optimism and perseverance in the therapy of Ankylosing Spondylitis. It emphasises how crucial it is to take a holistic approach that takes into account a person's emotional and psychological health in addition to the condition's outward symptoms. A more holistic view of health and wellness is made possible by recognising the connection between the body and mind.

We are faced with an interesting conundrum as we learn more about the complex interactions between Ankylosing Spondylitis and the body: How can we keep encouraging resilience and a sense of empowerment in the face of such difficulties? This inquiry acts as a lighthouse, pointing the way for additional research and interaction with the deeply intricate details of Ankylosing Spondylitis and its treatment.

Psychological and Emotional Effects

Set the Scene:

Imagine this: a peaceful morning with a warm glow emanating from a pleasant living room as the sun peeks through the curtains. A person sits in this calm area, lost in meditation as they battle the invisible burden of ankylosing spondylitis.

Introduce the Main Players:

Introducing Amelia, a vivacious person with an unquestionable love for life. Beneath her outward joy, though, she struggles with the emotional and psychological effects of having ankylosing spondylitis. Her trip is a deep investigation on resiliency and persistence.

Present the Challenge or Problem:

Amelia has to navigate the complex emotional web that comes with having ankylosing spondylitis, which is a challenging challenge. She faces a turbulent mental and emotional terrain as a result of the constant agony, the changing limits, and the unknown future.

Detail the Approach or Solution:

A multimodal approach is essential in addressing the psychological and emotional impacts of ankylosing spondylitis. Through individualised therapy, mindfulness exercises, and holistic approaches to wellness, Amelia sets out on a life-changing path toward resilience and emotional recovery.

Showcase the Results:

Significant changes start to happen in Amelia's life as the holistic healing strands spread. She finds deep strength reserves she was unaware of and her mental toughness blooms. The emotional terrain that was before turbulent becomes a calm haven of empowerment and self-acceptance.

Analyze and Reflect:

Amelia's journey case study highlights the significant influence of treating the psychological and emotional consequences of having ankylosing spondylitis. It emphasises the value of holistic wellness activities in fostering mental toughness and emotional stability, providing a ray of hope for those facing comparable difficulties.

Visual Aids (if applicable):

Imagine a soft visualisation that illustrates how emotions change from raging waves to calm seas, signifying the significant change in Amelia's emotional terrain.

Connect to the Larger Narrative or Concept:

Amelia's experience is a microcosm of the larger storey about managing ankylosing spondylitis. Understanding the complex relationship between mental and physical health opens the door to complete, holistic restoration.

Transition Thought or Question:

As we explore the intricacies of emotional health within the framework of Ankylosing Spondylitis, let us consider the following: How may the incorporation of holistic wellness techniques enhance the emotional terrain of those managing chronic illnesses?

We take a fascinating look at the psychological and emotional impacts of ankylosing spondylitis in this chapter. We discover the significant influence of holistic wellbeing on mental toughness and emotional stability via the prism of Amelia's experience. Come along with me as we untangle the complex web of emotions and create avenues for complete healing and self-determination.

Quality of Life Implications

Introduction to the Topic:

It is essential that we explore the complex web of ways that Ankylosing Spondylitis affects our day-to-day lives as we set out on this path to comprehend and control this condition. Ankylosing Spondylitis is more than simply a physical illness; it's a multifaceted force that affects every facet of our lives. This illness permeates all aspect of our life, affecting everything from our jobs to the way we love, our interests to our downtime.

State the Claim or Proposition:

This subchapter will address the assertion that Ankylosing Spondylitis has a significant impact on life quality across a range of domains, including work, relationships, and leisure activities.

Present Primary Evidence:

First, let's talk about how ankylosing spondylitis affects a person's ability to work. According to studies, people with Ankylosing Spondylitis frequently struggle to keep a job because of the physical restrictions placed on them by the illness. Ankylosing Spondylitis's persistent pain, stiffness, and exhaustion can seriously impair a person's performance in a regular work environment.

Delve Deeper into the Evidence:

Ankylosing Spondylitis discomfort and stiffness can make even the most straightforward work tasks seem impossible. People might therefore find it difficult to fulfil the obligations of their professions, which would result in lower productivity and higher absenteeism. Furthermore, juggling a career and a chronic illness can have a tremendous emotional toll, which increases stress and worry.

Counter-evidence or Counterarguments:

It is imperative to recognise that certain individuals suffering with Ankylosing Spondylitis are capable of securing employment accommodations that enable them to carry out their duties with efficiency. More supportive work settings have also been made possible by developments in the condition's awareness and treatment.

Rebuttal or Clarification:

Although accommodations and assistance can be very helpful, it's important to understand that many people still struggle greatly with the effects of ankylosing spondylitis on their ability to function in the workplace. Even with accommodations in place, the condition's unexpected nature and the symptoms' varying severity can make it challenging to regularly keep employment.

Additional Supporting Evidence (optional):

Ankylosing Spondylitis affects relationships and leisure activities in addition to the workplace. Because Ankylosing Spondylitis is a chronic ailment, relationships with spouses, family, and friends may be strained as they attempt to comprehend the day-to-day struggles that sufferers of the illness experience. Relationship quality may suffer as a result of this lack of understanding, which can also cause emotions of dissatisfaction and loneliness.

Conclusion with Reinforced Assertion:

In conclusion, there are many different aspects and ramifications of Ankylosing Spondylitis on day-to-day living. Even if there are times when people overcome obstacles and succeed, it's important to recognise how much this condition affects relationships, employment, and leisure activities. By being aware of these consequences, we can start to develop a thorough management strategy for ankylosing spondylitis that respects every aspect of our lives.

Medical Management of Ankylosing Spondylitis

Non-Steroidal Anti-Inflammatory Drugs (NSAIDs)

Welcome, reader, to the world of managing ankylosing spondylitis (AS), as we set out to comprehend and overcome the difficulties this condition presents. I, Dr. Ankita Kashyap, am delighted to be your guide and walk with you, providing empowering solutions and holistic insights to help you master the art of living well with AS.

Now, let's talk about Non-Steroidal Anti-Inflammatory Drugs (NSAIDs), which are essential for the treatment of AS. These drugs have the ability to reduce inflammation and ease discomfort, giving this condition some reprieve.

NSAIDs are an essential part of the therapeutic armament for AS since they help reduce the pain and stiffness that are frequently associated with the condition. These drugs provide a route to respite for people navigating the challenges of AS by preventing the body from producing chemicals that cause pain and inflammation.

One of the most important strategies for controlling the pain and inflammation brought on by ankylosing spondylitis is the use of NSAIDs.

Studies have shown that NSAIDs are effective in helping people with AS feel less painful and stiff. Studies and clinical trials have demonstrated how these drugs can help people who are struggling with the effects of AS move more easily and live better overall.

NSAIDs are not only useful for treating symptoms; they may also slow down the advancement of spinal inflammation in AS patients. NSAIDs act as protectors, preventing the problem from worsening and protecting the spine by targeting inflammation at its source.

Recognizing the possible negative effects of long-term NSAID use, such as gastrointestinal issues and cardiovascular concerns, is essential. These factors demand a careful approach to drug management and close coordination with medical professionals in order to weigh the advantages and disadvantages of NSAID therapy.

Although there is reason to be concerned about the possible adverse effects of NSAIDs, prudent usage and close observation can allay these worries. The dangers associated with NSAID therapy can be reduced by customising treatment plans and implementing preventative measures, enabling people to benefit from pain relief and inflammation control without suffering unnecessary consequences.

Research has demonstrated how NSAIDs can enhance function and decrease disease activity in AS, highlighting the many advantages of these drugs. Furthermore, improvements in pharmaceutical formulations have produced NSAIDs with better safety profiles, providing a promising future for people looking for treatment from symptoms associated with AS.

To sum up, the careful application of nonsteroidal anti-inflammatory drugs (NSAIDs) is a crucial tactic in the all-encompassing treatment of osteoarthritis (OSI). People with AS can traverse the terrain more easily and resiliently if they make the most of these drugs while being aware of any possible hazards. The ability to effectively administer NSAID medication is a ray of hope that illuminates the way to a life that is full of comfort and energy and that is not constrained by AS.

Let's embrace the knowledge and opportunities that lie ahead as we continue our investigation of AS management, creating a path towards empowerment and overall well-being. We set out on a journey together that is lighted by wisdom, empathy, and the steadfast spirit of resilience.

Disease-Modifying Antirheumatic Drugs (DMARDs)

Greetings, my love, and welcome to the amazing world of controlling ankylosing spondylitis. Here, we will set out on a path of comprehension, recovery, and self-determination. We explore the critical role that disease-modifying antirheumatic medications (DMARDs) play in the all-encompassing treatment of ankylosing spondylitis in this subchapter. Let's examine the subtleties of DMARDs as effective medications that can prevent joint damage and slow the course of this illness.

Imagine a calm, sunlit morning, a warm, golden light filling a small clinic space, and the comforting buzz of healing energy permeating the atmosphere. Here is where our storey begins, in a place where people seeking wellness join together with healthcare professionals in a refuge of hope and opportunity.

Here is our protagonist: a determined person battling Ankylosing Spondylitis and looking for answers and comfort among the confusing array of medical possibilities. Beside them, an empathetic group of medical specialists, including myself, Dr. Ankita Kashyap, and a committed group of experts from several domains, who are all committed to the goal of holistic therapy.

The terrifying possibility of Ankylosing Spondylitis, a disorder marked by inflammation and stiffness in the spine and joints, is faced by our main character. Even the most basic daily activities are threatened by the disease's unrelenting advance, which poses a threat to their quality of life. It becomes imperative to stop it from getting worse and lessen joint damage—a problem that still needs to be solved.

A family of drugs called DMARDs, which are intended to alter the course of inflammatory disorders, appears as a ray of hope in this developing drama. These medications, with their diverse processes, are prepared to provide relief and respite to individuals suffering from

Ankylosing Spondylitis. We negotiate the maze of DMARD choices by means of meticulous evaluation and individualised treatment strategies, customising each strategy to meet the specific requirements and goals of our protagonist.

The impact of DMARDs becomes evident as the narrative progresses, creating a tapestry of advancement and hope. Joint damage is reduced, the unrelenting march of inflammation is subdued, and the once-elusive feeling of freedom and mobility starts to emerge through the haze of doubt. Savoring the wonderful taste of vitality, our protagonist retrieves happy and spontaneous moments that were previously believed to have been lost to the clutches of Ankylosing Spondylitis.

In the middle of the victories and discoveries, we take a moment to learn from this storey of resiliency and rejuvenation. We reflect on the fine balance that exists between science and empathy, the skill of customising care to respect each patient's unique needs, and the persistent need to push the boundaries of wellness research. However, we continue to be aware of any objections, realising that every trip is as distinct as a fingerprint and that there are many facets to the healing process.

Visual aids act as windows into learning throughout this trip, providing glimpses into the complex mechanics at work within the human body. These visual aids, which range from tasteful diagrams that illustrate how DMARDs work to moving before-and-after pictures, enhance our storey and encourage greater attention and understanding.

This storey of success and metamorphosis fits into the larger picture of managing ankylosing spondylitis—a monument to the efficacy of fusing conventional knowledge with state-of-the-art research. It touches on the core of our main issue, which is the significant role that individualised, comprehensive treatment plays in helping patients navigate the maze of chronic illness.

Let us ponder the following question as we bid adieu to this captivating storey: What more gems lie in store for discovery in the field of managing ankylosing spondylitis? We go out with the hope that DMARDs will provide us with a beacon of light, always inquisitive and ready to discover the plethora of opportunities that lie ahead.

We have hardly touched on the vast influence of DMARDs on the field of managing ankylosing spondylitis in this subchapter. Come along as we explore the depths of holistic healing, peel back the layers of this engrossing storey, and illuminate the road to empowerment and well-being.

Biological Therapies

Greetings, reader, and welcome to an investigation into the intriguing realm of biological treatments for the treatment of Ankylosing Spondylitis. This subchapter will take us on a tour of the complex world of TNF inhibitors, IL-17 inhibitors, and IL-23 inhibitors and reveal their significant influence on the management of this illness. Now let us set off on this magical journey where science and hope mingle and healing meets possibilities.

Imagine a patient, Sarah, attempting to navigate the maze-like anguish and discomfort that ankylosing spondylitis frequently brings. Once upon a time, Sarah's days were marred by a constant aching in her back, tight joints, and a persistent fatigue that followed her around like a shadow. When she went in search of care, she came upon the field of biological therapies, which was full of hope for recovery and alleviation.

Throughout Sarah's journey, the amazing biological therapies—each with a unique storey to tell—had a crucial part. The mysterious TNF inhibitors arose as formidable defenders, bucking the inflammatory wave that threatened to consume Sarah's life force. Then the elusive IL-17 inhibitors appeared, delicately encircling her joints in a protective net to keep them safe from the devastation caused by Ankylosing Spondylitis. Not to be outdone, her immune system was protected by the gallant IL-23 inhibitors, which stepped in to maintain its delicate balance in the face of the inflammatory storm.

Sarah had challenges not just in her physical health but also in her emotional and mental health. The obstacles that loomed big were the unknown, the feeling of being imprisoned by her own body, and the fear of what was ahead. It was becoming more and more obvious that she needed a treatment that could not only make her bodily symptoms better but also give her a sense of confidence and empowerment.

Step inside the fascinating realm of biological therapeutics, where empathy and science came together to provide a solution that went beyond simple symptom control. Sarah's inflammation decreased, her pain lessened, and her energy returned with a customised prescription of TNF inhibitors. The chivalrous IL-17 inhibitors worked their magic, restoring mobility to her joints, while the gallant IL-23 inhibitors preserved her immunological equilibrium, protecting her from the unpleasant embrace of disease development.

Sarah's life underwent a shift that could only be described as amazing. She began to emerge from the boundaries of her discomfort as the biological therapies took hold, flowering into a fresh sense of possibilities and freedom. With every day that went by, the burden of her illness lessened and she came to embrace the once-elusive joys of mobility and activity. The visible effects of these therapies shone through the prism of facts and firsthand accounts, revealing the way back to a life recovered.

We are encouraged to consider the important lessons buried within Sarah's tale as we observe her trip. The striking efficacy of biologic therapy suggests a paradigm change in the treatment of ankylosing spondylitis that goes beyond the constraints of conventional methods. Even so, in the middle of this joy, we must continue to be aware of any objections and difficulties, realising the necessity of further study and improvement in this amazing field of healing.

Visual aids appear as soft guides inside the fabric of Sarah's storey, providing us with hints about the complex mechanisms underlying biological therapies. These visual cues inspire us to explore the field of healing further because they portray a picture of optimism and possibilities. Examples of these cues include the graceful dancing of molecules, the subtle changes in inflammation, and the graceful modulation of immune responses.

The storey of Sarah is a beautiful thread that is woven into the overall picture of managing ankylosing spondylitis. By means of her experiences, we are invited to consider the astounding possibilities of biological therapies—not just as cures but as agents of change. Their influence extends beyond the person, striking at the core of holistic health and the desire to live free from the constraints of disease.

A question that keeps coming to mind as we say goodbye to Sarah's fascinating trip is like a soft melody: what more secrets and wonders are in wait for us in the field of biological therapies? Allow this query to pique your interest and create a desire to learn more about this fascinating field of hope and healing.

We have only scratched the surface of the fascinating world of biological therapies in this subchapter, but there are hints of promise and opportunity all around us, beckoning us to continue our search for enlightenment and a deeper understanding. As we say our goodbyes, may the sound of Sarah's journey resound inside you, igniting awe and curiosity that leads you on your own journey of self-discovery and mastery.

Physical Therapy and Rehabilitation

: Unlocking the Power of Movement

Physical therapy and rehabilitation become an invaluable ally as we navigate the complex maze of managing ankylosing spondylitis. Imagine yourself in a calm space bathed in the mild light of dawn as a series of calming, revitalising movements take place. Here, in the perfect symphony of peace and resolve, is where movement's transformational power resides.

Envision, if you will, the tale of an extraordinary person, whom we shall refer to as Maya. Maya has been steadfast in the face of extreme obstacles as she navigates the maze of ankylosing spondylitis. The hope and resiliency that characterise her path seem to be echoed in the air as she enters the world of physical therapy and rehabilitation.

Our main characters in this storey are Maya and Sarah, her devoted physical therapist. Maya, a source of steadfast fortitude, has been battling Ankylosing Spondylitis's limitations and longs to regain the mobility she once loved. Sarah, a seasoned physical therapy advisor, crafts individualised plans to support Maya's journey to wellness with a wealth of knowledge and compassion.

Maya faces a powerful opponent on her path to recovery: the omnipresent grip of stiffness and restricted movement. Her dreams of leading a full and active life are frequently threatened by the sneaky vines of agony and suffering that gnaw at her soul.

Step into the world of physical therapy, where each session is a mosaic of conscious movements, mild stretches, and targeted exercises. Sarah creates a customised strategy that is painstakingly adjusted to Maya's particular requirements. She uses endurance, strength, and flexibility to overcome the limitations imposed by Ankylosing Spondylitis. Every aspect of this mosaic, including yoga, pilates, and water therapy, has the potential to release Maya and help her body find its flowing grace.

Maya's burgeoning vigour is bursting from the tendrils of stiffness that unravel with every session that goes by. Her steps become more confident and flowing, and the radiant smile that lights up her face belies the freedom she has discovered. The measurements of improvement, which are a concrete reflection of her commitment, offer a striking picture of change: greater mobility in the spine, less discomfort, and a vigour that goes beyond figures.

Looking at this storey of recovery, we can learn a great deal about the complex relationship between physical therapy and Ankylosing Spondylitis. It invites us to consider the nuanced relationship between recovery and resilience, the alchemical union of spirit and science that forms the basis of healing arts. However, even as we recognise Maya's accomplishments, we are also struck by the complex web of difficulties that still permeates the lives of innumerable people living with this illness.

Imagine a sequence of soft, poetic drawings that capture the spirit of each healing exercise: the flowing line of a yoga position, the calm of swimming therapy, and the unwavering will that propels these pursuits. Allow these graphic tales to convey a message of peace and optimism, enticing the reader to experience the life-changing power of movement.

Physical therapy and rehabilitation play a significant role in the overall management of Ankylosing Spondylitis, as they signal a return to mobility and vigour. They invite us to consider the profoundly positive relationship that exists between movement therapy and holistic wellbeing, as well as to embrace a paradigm in which the body, mind, and spirit work together in harmonious union.

A poignant question remains unanswered as we continue to follow Maya's journey: what other unsung stories of resiliency and healing are waiting to be revealed within the supportive environment of physical therapy and rehabilitation? Allow this query to pique your interest and ignite a desire to discover the countless transformational stories that are just waiting to be discovered, providing insights into the tremendous potential of movement as a healing medium.

We set off on a journey through the bright landscapes of physical therapy and rehabilitation, with the soothing rhythm of Maya's storey resonating in our hearts. Every step we take becomes a monument to the persevering spirit that survives amidst the maze of Ankylosing Spondylitis.

Exercise and Stretching

Greetings from the world of movement, where the secrets of power, flexibility, and vitality are whispered by your body. We will go on an exploration of the transforming potential of stretching and exercise in addressing the difficulties associated with Ankylosing Spondylitis in this chapter. By working together, we will discover the secret of movement, opening doors to increased joint health, flexibility, and symptom relief. Will you join me in embracing the dance of wellness? Now let's get started.

Our goal is to provide our bodies a sense of independence and resilience by utilising the therapeutic power of consistent exercise and stretching to lessen the effects of Ankylosing Spondylitis.

All you need to start this journey is an open heart, a readiness to pay attention to your body, and a dedication to taking care of your physical health. The only necessities are comfy clothes, a secure area to move around, and maybe a gentle reminder to take deep breaths.

Picture a gentle symphony, with every movement representing a note in the song of health. To begin, let's review the fundamentals of stretching and exercising and see how they could help reduce the stiffness and pain that come with having ankylosing spondylitis. After that, we'll get into certain workouts and stretches designed to support and foster your individual journey.

Let's start our investigation with soft motions that respect the body's natural desire for elegance and flow. Pilates, yoga, and tai chi provide a balanced combination of strength, flexibility, and awareness; they are kind allies in your journey to well-being. Next, we'll explore the world of stretching, where each lengthening of a muscle fibre turns into a gentle act of self-care. You will be able to recover your range of motion by adopting a stretching regimen that include both passive and vigorous stretching.

It is imperative that you pay attention to your body's whispers as we set out on this life-changing trip. Honor the feedback from your muscles and the rhythm of your breath as you begin slowly. To guarantee that your exercises are customised to your specific requirements, seek advice from a certified fitness specialist. Remember that patience is the softest virtue on this path, and be aware of whatever pain or suffering you may be experiencing.

How can we tell whether the movement in our dance is producing the desired results? The beauty is in the small moments when your comfort zone opens up, the calm moments when your body feels at ease, and the newfound strength you have while facing stiffness. As your joints grow more flexible and your movements more fluid, you will experience the subtle harmony of personal development.

If you experience periods of discomfort or resistance, go back and review the basic principles of movement. Maybe your body is aching for a different kind of exercise or a kinder way to stretch. Pay great attention and be receptive to the small cues that lead you to a more harmonic connection with movement.

Let us keep in mind as we wrap up this chapter that movement is a meaningful dialogue with the body, mind, and spirit rather than just a sequence of physical acts. Open your heart to the trip and let each step create a healing tapestry inside of you.

We shall explore nutrition's therapeutic potential and how it can support your body's natural resilience in the upcoming chapter. May you have calm breathing, graceful movements, and a spirit filled with well-being until then.

Surgical Interventions

Greetings, reader, and welcome to this crucial juncture in our exploration of the complex world of managing ankylosing spondylitis. As we make our way through the complex maze of chronic illness, we come to a crucial intersection where human spirit and medical expertise collide. Today, we explore the world of surgical procedures, where brave individuals overcoming the difficulties of Ankylosing Spondylitis may find relief and a newfound sense of transformation.

Let's sketch out the current situation before we set out on this investigation. With its sneaky hold on the spine and joints of the body, ankylosing spondylitis frequently poses severe obstacles that are resistant to standard medical interventions. Even though we strongly believe in the benefits of holistic medicine and wellness, there are situations in which surgical procedures become lifelines for those suffering from serious joint damage and spinal issues.

The main problem we face is that Ankylosing Spondylitis progresses over time and can result in spinal fusion and irreparable joint damage. The quality of life declines and the capacity to carry out everyday tasks is increasingly affected as the illness worsens.

The effects of advanced Ankylosing Spondylitis might be severe if treatment is not received. For patients suffering with this disorder, abnormalities in the spine and joints, restricted movement, and chronic discomfort may become unwelcome companions. Such physical problems have an emotional and psychological cost that is incalculable since they undermine people's resilience and spirit.

Despite these overwhelming obstacles, surgical procedures provide a glimmer of hope. For those with advanced Ankylosing Spondylitis, joint replacement surgery and spinal fusion are two important treatments that have the potential to improve overall quality of life, relieve pain, and restore function.

Thinking about having joint replacement surgery? The procedure entails carefully removing worn-out joint surfaces and replacing them with synthetic parts. Through painless, painless joint restoration, patients will be able to move freely again and take up their regular activities with fresh energy after this painstaking operation.

In contrast, spinal fusion entails the union of two or more vertebrae in the spine in order to stabilise the afflicted joints and relieve discomfort that arises from their movement. This surgery seeks to provide a firm foundation for the spine and alleviate pain by solidifying the union between the vertebrae and preventing additional damage.

The life-changing effects of these surgical therapies on patients with advanced Ankylosing Spondylitis have been extensively documented, and multiple success stories attest to their usefulness. For individuals who have persevered through the tempest of this illness, these therapies hold the promise of a new chapter of life and freedom, from the restoration of movement to the relief of chronic pain.

Although surgical procedures present attractive opportunities for patients with severe joint deterioration and spinal problems, complementary therapies including physical therapy, pharmaceutical management, and lifestyle modifications remain vital in the overall management of Ankylosing Spondylitis. These options meet the multifaceted needs of people on their path to wellbeing in a perfect symphony of care when combined with surgical treatments.

It's critical to view these possibilities with a combination of caution and optimism as we continue to piece together the surgical procedures for Ankylosing Spondylitis. Since every person's journey is different, choosing to pursue surgical interventions should be based on a careful analysis of the advantages, possible risks, and specific factors.

We will go into further detail about the specifics of getting ready for and recuperating from surgical procedures in the upcoming chapter, giving you the information and self-assurance you need to get through this life-changing stage of your Ankylosing Spondylitis journey. Let the prospect of rejuvenation and restoration guide you on your journey of exploration until then.

In the field of managing ankylosing spondylitis, healing takes many forms, all of which are infused with hope and resiliency. Let us approach this path with reverence, inquiry, and an unshakable devotion to the great art of holistic wellbeing as we embrace the transforming possibilities of surgical treatments.

Complementary and Alternative Medicine

Greetings from the fascinating field of complementary and alternative medicine (CAM), where cutting-edge research and age-old knowledge converge to provide a comprehensive approach to health. Imagine a peaceful garden where the soft breeze whispers about herbal treatments and the soothing touch of acupuncture needles dances down the pathways of vitality, as we set off on this exploration. In order to help you embrace a symphony of healing modalities that speak to your body, mind, and spirit, we will be revealing here the possible advantages of complementary and alternative medicine (CAM) in managing the many nuances of ankylosing spondylitis.

To handle Ankylosing Spondylitis completely, we must take into account the amazing benefits of complementary and alternative medicine. Conventional medical interventions are important, but complementary and alternative medicine (CAM) offers a healing tapestry that can complement conventional treatments and support a holistic approach to wellness. Come, let's stroll through the lush meadows of CAM, where every medicinal bloom promises relief and rejuvenation.

Summarizing the main idea of our investigation, we claim that complementary and alternative medicine (CAM), which includes practises like acupuncture, herbal medicines, and mind-body approaches, has the potential to reduce the symptoms of Ankylosing Spondylitis and aid in its management. This is not just a whimsical tangent; rather, it is a statement supported by verifiable data that has been painstakingly assembled from the vast array of empirical research and scientific knowledge.

Acupuncture is our first introduction to the fascinating world of complementary and alternative medicine. Acupuncture, as subtle as a cherry flower and as deep as a mountain torrent, stimulates particular sites along the body's meridian pathways in an effort to bring back vitality and balance. According to studies, acupuncture may be a helpful ally in your quest for comfort and resilience by reducing the pain and inflammation linked to ankylosing spondylitis.

By looking more closely at the data, we are able to understand the complex processes that acupuncture uses to potentially heal. It is thought that stimulating acupuncture sites alters the neuroendocrine system of the body, causing endorphins and other neuropeptides with strong analgesic and anti-inflammatory effects to be released. Additionally, it is believed that acupuncture controls immunological responses, which may have an impact on the underlying inflammatory processes associated with ankylosing spondylitis. These results offer strong evidence for the potential of acupuncture as an adjunctive treatment for Ankylosing Spondylitis.

While we savour the calm radiance of acupuncture's possibilities, we must recognise the rich diversity of viewpoints that enhance our comprehension. There are legitimate worries or doubts expressed by some about the effectiveness of acupuncture in treating ankylosing spondylitis. Their counterarguments could come from the fact that more convincing clinical proof is needed or from the fact that each person's reaction to acupuncture is different. In response to these objections, however, we are reassured by the increasing amount of evidence demonstrating the potential benefits of acupuncture for the treatment of inflammatory diseases such as Ankylosing Spondylitis and pain.

Herbal remedies flourish with the rich hues of old therapeutic traditions in the verdant environment of complementary and alternative medicine. Herbal medicines, ranging from the soft whispers of chamomile to the strong hug of turmeric, provide a wealth of botanical friends in the treatment of Ankylosing Spondylitis. The abundance of phytochemicals, each with distinct qualities that may boost immunological resilience, lessen inflammation, and ease pain are the main sources of evidence for the possible advantages of herbal therapies for ankylosing spondylitis.

Entering the aromatic realm of herbal medicines, we come across the vibrant colours of curcumin, the key ingredient in turmeric that is well-known for its strong anti-inflammatory qualities. Research findings indicate that curcumin could potentially regulate the inflammatory processes linked to Ankylosing Spondylitis, providing a herbal ray of hope in the face of persistent pain and inflammation. Moreover, the soft murmurs of herbal companions like ginger and Boswellia serrata promise to ease discomfort and build resilience.

Recognizing the counterarguments that raise doubts is crucial as we navigate the aromatic garden of herbal treatments. Regarding the possibility of herb-drug interactions as well as the standardisation and quality control of herbal products, scepticism may surface. But these worries can be allayed by using herbal therapies sparingly and under the supervision of trained medical specialists, guaranteeing a safe and seamless integration into the overall management of ankylosing spondylitis.

Similar to a peaceful pool reflecting the sky, mind-body therapies provide a significant means of fostering emotional fortitude and reducing the negative effects of stress on ankylosing spondylitis. Mind-body activities range widely, from the soft waves of mindfulness meditation to the elegant motions of tai chi. They challenge you to develop balance in the complex terrain of your being.

Research has demonstrated how mind-body practises can help people with Ankylosing Spondylitis feel better emotionally, move more easily, and have less discomfort. For example, practising mindfulness meditation gently might improve coping mechanisms and reduce psychological discomfort, providing a peaceful haven in the face of chronic illness. For those juggling the challenges of Ankylosing Spondylitis, the flowing motions of tai chi and yoga may also help with flexibility, balance, and general quality of life.

We recognise the arguments that could surface while we're submerging ourselves in the peaceful waters of mind-body practises.

While some may doubt the viability or accessibility of mind-body therapies, others may look for factual proof to support their possible advantages in the treatment of Ankylosing Spondylitis. But an increasing amount of studies and first-hand accounts highlight the significant benefits of mind-body practises in fostering resilience and overall wellbeing, providing a strong basis for their incorporation into the care of Ankylosing Spondylitis.

Within the soft embrace of complementary and alternative medicine, we have explored the enchanted paths of acupuncture, herbal medicines, and mind-body practises, each of which has a distinct therapeutic song that speaks to the complex subtleties of ankylosing spondylitis. As we draw to a close, the harmony of data and practical knowledge supports the claim that complementary and alternative medicine (CAM) has the ability to assist in the management of rheumatoid arthritis (AS) by creating a healing mosaic that is in harmony with conventional medical interventions.

I hope that this window into the world of complementary and alternative medicine will pique your interest and inspire you to set out on a path to well-being that combines the knowledge of cutting-edge research with the wisdom of age-old healing practises. CAM is a gentle ally in the verdant garden of managing ankylosing spondylitis, providing a tapestry of therapeutic techniques that align with the delicate harmony of your being.

Holistic Approaches to Ankylosing Spondylitis Management

The Role of Nutrition in Ankylosing Spondylitis

Title: Nutrition's Significance in Ankylosing Spondylitis: Nourishing Your Body, Nurturing Your Health

Welcome to a universe where the experience of Ankylosing Spondylitis collides with the power of nutrition. As we go out on this journey together, I cordially ask you to be open-minded and receptive to the significant influence that your diet has on your overall health. Let's examine the complex relationship between food and inflammation and how our experience with Ankylosing Spondylitis might be influenced by the decisions we make at the dinner table.

Our bodies are magnificent temples, with a vibrant community of cells vying for balance and harmony within each one. The importance of diet is paramount in the world of Ankylosing Spondylitis, where inflammation is the norm and pain can be an unwanted guest. Here, we explore the maze of nourishment and examine how food may be calming, restorative, and energising.

Today, we will examine the assertion that diet has a significant influence on the treatment of ankylosing spondylitis. We suggest that addressing food sensitivities, implementing strategic supplements, and implementing an anti-inflammatory diet can have a revolutionary effect on the management of this condition's symptoms and progression.

Let's start by discussing the fundamentals of an anti-inflammatory diet. Studies indicate that some foods have a remarkable capacity to suppress inflammation in the body. It has been demonstrated that foods high in omega-3 fatty acids, like walnuts, flaxseeds, and fatty fish, have anti-inflammatory properties. In addition, adding colourful fruits and vegetables—especially those that are loaded with antioxidants and color—can supply vital nutrients and fight oxidative stress, which is a typical symptom of Ankylosing Spondylitis.

Think about the common blueberry, a small yet powerful friend in the fight against inflammation. These little jewels, bursting with anthocyanins, have strong anti-inflammatory qualities. Imagine the rich, deep colours of a ripe blueberry, and picture this organic powerhouse enveloping your body in its protective shell. You may strengthen your body against the damaging effects of inflammation and entice your taste buds by include such fruits in your regular diet.

Let's now move our focus to the supplements industry. The attraction of supplements is their ability to provide our systems with specific nutrients. Some supplements may be able to help people with Ankylosing Spondylitis manage their symptoms and maintain their general health. In addition to its well-known function in maintaining bone health, vitamin D has drawn interest for its capacity to control immunological responses and lower inflammation. Examining the sun vitamin, we find that it has a complex relationship with our immune system and provides a glimmer of hope for managing Ankylosing Spondylitis.

Divergent opinions frequently compete for attention in the field of nutrition. Some may argue that because illness processes are complex, food has little bearing on inflammatory disorders. Recognizing the intricacies involved and the unique differences in our bodies' responses to dietary changes is crucial.

We cannot ignore the strong body of evidence indicating the involvement of nutrition in inflammatory disorders, even though the relationship between nutrition and health is complex. The intricate relationship between our diet and the inflammatory pathways in our bodies is a complex web that may have an impact on how Ankylosing Spondylitis is treated.

Expanding on our investigation, we come across the domain of dietary sensitivities. Some people with Ankylosing Spondylitis may experience increased immune reactions in response to specific meals, which can exacerbate inflammation and symptoms. People can create a dietary landscape that reduces possible triggers and promotes a kinder relationship with their bodies by recognising and managing these sensitivities.

We find ourselves at the brink of potential as we close the door on our exploration. The importance of diet in Ankylosing Spondylitis is evidence of the close relationship between food and health. By implementing an anti-inflammatory diet, strategically using supplements, and carefully navigating food sensitivities, people can utilise nutrition as a fundamental component in their journey towards effectively controlling and prospering from Ankylosing Spondylitis.

We go deeper into the skill of creating a supporting and nourishing connection with food in the pages that follow, providing you with a tapestry of flavours, insights, and guidance to enhance your journey. Accept the transforming potential of diet, and allow food's ability to heal to become a valued ally in your quest to conquer ankylosing spondylitis.

Exercise and Movement Therapy

Welcome to the life-changing process of managing your Ankylosing Spondylitis with exercise and movement therapy. We will explore the effectiveness of particular exercises and movement therapies in this subchapter, giving you a comprehensive plan for pain management, posture correction, and general well-being.

Our goal is to provide you with a step-by-step action plan that will not only reduce the pain that comes with having ankylosing spondylitis but also enable you to take back control of your body and mind by using specific movement and exercise regimens.

You must have an open mind, be willing to accept change, and be determined to put your health and wellbeing first in order to start this journey. In order to improve comfort and safety, several activities may also just need basic equipment like yoga mats, resistance bands, or supportive cushions.

We will begin by discussing the various forms of exercise and movement therapies that have proven to be quite beneficial for people with Ankylosing Spondylitis. We'll cover a range of techniques that suit different needs and interests, from mind-body activities like yoga and tai chi to light stretching and strengthening exercises.

Let's start with some mild stretching exercises to assist increase flexibility and decrease stiffness. These movements focus on the hips, chest, and spine. After that, we'll switch to strengthening activities that target the back and core muscles in an effort to improve the stability and support of the spine. After that, we will practise yoga and tai chi to further explore the mind-body connection while promoting better posture, relaxation, and awareness.

Remember to pay attention to your body's signals and respect its limitations when you perform these exercises and movement therapies. Work your way through the exercises gradually, letting yourself settle into a rhythm that is both energising and cosy. Seek advice from a skilled expert to make sure the workouts are customised to your unique requirements and skill level. Furthermore, pay attention to any warning indications, such as heightened pain or discomfort, and modify the technique or intensity as needed.

When you start to feel more mobile, have less pain and stiffness, have better posture, and generally feel better about yourself, you've successfully incorporated exercise and movement therapy into your routine. These progress indicators will confirm the beneficial effects these techniques are having on your Ankylosing Spondylitis journey.

Don't give up if you run into difficulties or setbacks along the road. As you set out on a new journey of self-care and healing, it is normal to encounter challenges. Always remember to be open and honest with your medical team, ask for help from other people who also have Ankylosing Spondylitis, and look into different exercise regimens that might be more appropriate for your particular situation.

Imagine each movement you perform as a gentle dance between your body and the healing energy that surrounds you as you immerse yourself in the world of fitness and movement therapy. Accept the flow of your breath as you lengthen, fortify, and move; you are nourishing your body and soul with each intentional movement.

Discover the bliss of motion, the peace of quiet, and the close relationship between your body and mind. As you set out on this revolutionary journey towards comprehensive well-being, allow your heart's rhythm to lead the way.

I hope this section acts as a lighthouse of inspiration, sparking a fresh understanding of your body's amazing potential and the healing effects of movement. As you gently enrich your days with movement therapy and exercise, accept each moment with grace and thankfulness.

We will go into even more complementary techniques and self-care practises in the pages that follow, which will enhance your experience and take your Ankylosing Spondylitis management to the next level of mastery.

Allow the healing process to happen, and may the beat of wellness bring comfort to your soul.

Warm regards,

Dr. Ankita Kashyap

Stress Management and Relaxation Techniques

Welcome to the peaceful haven of stress relief and relaxation methods, where you can feel the comforting embrace of peace and soft murmurs of tranquilly. We will set out on a journey to investigate the profound effects of mindfulness, deep breathing techniques, and meditation on the complex fabric of managing ankylosing spondylitis in this tranquil refuge. Let us unfold these techniques' delicate petals to reveal the magnificent bloom of holistic well-being they offer.

Imagine a calm garden where the sound of rustling leaves combines with the melodious sounds of nature, all surrounded by the golden glow of the setting sun. In this beautiful environment, we meet Sarah—a brilliant person who struggles with the crippling effects of ankylosing spondylitis. The pain that never goes away from her joints and the exhaustion that pulls at her soul cast a cloud on her days.

Sarah has set out on a mission to recover her vitality and find the joy of life. She is a strong, unwavering spirit. Beside her is an empathetic group of health and wellness professionals, guided steadfastly by Dr. Ankita Kashyap, a proponent of holistic healing and wellbeing. By combining their expertise and support from several sectors, they create a tapestry that gives Sarah a comprehensive approach to her journey.

The main obstacle that Sarah must overcome is the constant stress in her life. Stress clouds her days and makes her ankylosing spondylitis worse. She is surrounded by a cocoon of sorrow as the weight of her suffering and the load of her doubt create a tangled web.

Sarah and her team of professionals explore the calm world of stress management and relaxation techniques in response to this difficult issue. They set out on a quest to discover the profound art of awareness, the calming rhythm of deep breathing exercises, and the transformational power of meditation. They collaborate to create a customised strategy that integrates these methods into Sarah's everyday activities.

Sarah discovers herself engulfed in the peace of these activities as the days go by. The noise of tension starts to fade, and the strands of calmness slowly unfurl inside her. The dull pain that had imprisoned her starts to loosen, and exhaustion's pressure starts to lessen. Once an uncommon sight, Sarah's smile now brightens her way like a beautiful flower.

We get a deep understanding of the transformational power of stress reduction and relaxation practises via the lens of Sarah's journey. The subtle magic of these exercises has not only lifted the weight of stress but also rippled through Sarah's life, giving it a fresh lease on life and resiliency. It is imperative to recognise that the effectiveness of these methods may differ for every person, and that their full potential is only fully achieved when integrated into a comprehensive management strategy for ankylosing spondylitis.

The reader is guided through the essentials of stress management and relaxation techniques in the peaceful haven of this subchapter by visual aids in the form of soothing imagery and soft graphics.

In the larger storey of managing ankylosing spondylitis, the fine threads of stress reduction and relaxation are essential components of overall health and wellbeing. They provide a haven of solace, enabling people to face the intricacies of their illness with dignity and fortitude.

While basking in the tranquillity, let us consider: How can the subtle art of stress reduction and relaxation techniques be further woven into the holistic healthcare system, providing comfort and empowerment to individuals navigating the maze of chronic illnesses?

May these methods be like lights in the soft tide that gently rises and falls on our journey, showing us the way to calm and wellness.

Sleep Optimization

As night falls and the world stills down, our bodies get ready for slumber's healing embrace. But for individuals enduring the difficult path of Ankylosing Spondylitis, getting a good night's sleep can seem like a far-off dream. It is impossible to overestimate the influence sleep problems have on managing the symptoms of Ankylosing Spondylitis. This subsection will examine the importance of getting a good night's sleep as well as doable tactics for improving sleep hygiene and managing sleep disruptions. So let's set off on this calming trip, my dear readers, to recover the serenity of sound sleep.

The value of getting enough good sleep is sometimes overlooked in the rush of contemporary living. On the other hand, sleep disturbances can have more serious repercussions for those who have Ankylosing Spondylitis. Sleep deprivation can intensify pain and inflammation, resulting in increased discomfort and limited range of motion. The negative effects of sleep deprivation on mental health are also undeniable, and managing this illness is made more difficult by increased weariness and mood swings.

The main problem at hand is how common sleep disorders are in people with ankylosing spondylitis. These disruptions, which range from trouble falling asleep to numerous nighttime awakenings to the sensation of unrefreshing sleep, lead to a vicious cycle of discomfort and a lowered quality of life. Its negative effects on one's mental and physical health should not be understated.

If these sleep disruptions are not addressed, people with Ankylosing Spondylitis may end up stuck in a vicious cycle of worsening symptoms. Increased stiffness and pain could make it harder to move about and make you feel more frustrated. Physical and mental exhaustion can become crippling, affecting day-to-day functioning and general well-being. Inadequate sleep has cumulative repercussions that can negatively impact all facets of an individual's life.

Prioritizing sleep optimization is crucial for Ankylosing Spondylitis management in order to break free from this cycle. People may improve symptom management and general well-being by putting specific sleep hygiene and sleep disruption management practises into practise.

Start by creating a relaxing bedtime ritual. Give your body a cue to relax by doing soothing exercises like mindful meditation, light stretching, or reading a book. Reduce light and noise in your bedroom, and buy pillows and mattresses that are comfortable and suit your body's specific demands to create a peaceful sleeping environment. To help you settle into a pleasant state of rest, you should also think about including relaxation techniques like progressive muscle relaxation or deep breathing exercises.

Given that pain has a significant impact on sleep, it's critical to collaborate closely with your healthcare team to successfully manage discomfort. To reduce pain and encourage relaxation, this may entail the use of specific drugs, physical therapy, or alternative therapies. Additionally, learning about the possible advantages of cognitive behavioural therapy for insomnia (CBT-I) can give people useful tools to treat the psychological causes of sleep disorders.

People with Ankylosing Spondylitis should expect a significant increase in their capacity to control their symptoms if they prioritise sleep optimization. Increased resilience in the face of everyday obstacles, elevated mood, and decreased pain perception have all been related to better sleep quality. People may discover that, with a restored sense of vitality and well-being, they are better able to manage the difficulties of this condition as the restorative power of sleep is harnessed.

Although the aforementioned tactics are important cornerstones of optimising sleep, it's important to understand that every person will react differently to interventions. There are more options for individualised sleep improvement when looking into alternate approaches, such as using wearable technology for sleep tracking or incorporating natural sleep aids. It's critical to approach sleep optimization with an open mind and embrace a wide range of solutions that are customised to meet each person's specific needs.

As we explore the peaceful world of sleep optimization, let's not forget that everyone has a unique route to sound sleep. Accepting the delicate practise of tending to our sleep lays the groundwork for a happier, more energetic life. Thus, my dear readers, may the calming embrace of a sound sleep lead the way to a revitalised feeling of health and energy.

Heat and Cold Therapies

We come across a multitude of methods and resources that come together to create the holistic wellness tapestry as we navigate the maze of Ankylosing Spondylitis. Among these, the traditional treatments of heat and cold serve as steadfast protectors, providing a break from the unrelenting waves of discomfort and inflammation. Let's investigate these straightforward yet effective treatments, exploring their subtleties and discovering the game-changing potential they have for managing ankylosing spondylitis.

Imagine yourself in a warm, well-lit space that is permeated with a soft, peaceful murmur. A patient suffering from Ankylosing Spondylitis sits in the centre of this peaceful area, trying to find relief from the unwavering hold of stiffness and pain. The wisdom of heat and cold therapies guides the healing process, and the air is filled with hopeful expectancy.

Introducing Sarah, a vibrant individual whose life has been entangled in the complications of having ankylosing spondylitis. Her steadfast will and boundless enthusiasm for life drove her to look for holistic medical care, which brought her to our healing haven. Beside her, the skilled hands of our wellness specialists, each a master in their field, are prepared to weave a fabric of relaxation and renewal.

The main obstacle we face is the constant pain and inflammation that Ankylosing Spondylitis patients must endure. How can we help people in need while navigating these turbulent waters? This is the enigma that calls us to solve its secrets.

We find our allies in the embrace of heat and cold therapy. Warm packs gently relieve the tension in tired muscles, promoting a feeling of ease and relaxation. They are like warm whispers of consolation. Cold compresses, like fresh, energising breaths of mountain air, give irritated joints a calming numbness that smothers the flaming talons of pain.

As these age-old remedies are carefully administered, Sarah feels her body's tensed defences gently loosening. Pain's unwavering hold relaxes, and inflammation's raging embers cool down to a soothing slumber. A picture of peace in the middle of the storm is painted by the symphony of relief that plays out.

We are invited to consider the tremendous simplicity of heat and cold therapies as we look at this therapeutic vignette. Their modest appearance betrays the profound effect they have, acting as pillars of support amidst the turbulent waters of Ankylosing Spondylitis. Even in the midst of their soft embrace, these therapies are merely modest instruments in the vast scheme of holistic healing, so we must continue to be watchful and alert.

Imagine the symphony of relief and renewal that is woven by the delicate dance of warmth and cooling. Allow the images of these treatments to fill you with calm and relaxation.

The threads of heat and cold therapy are subtle yet effective relief agents in the larger picture of managing ankylosing spondylitis. Their existence serves as evidence of the enormous benefits of simplicity and serves as a reminder that, despite healthcare's intricacies, sometimes the most basic instruments have the most power.

While we bask in the warmth of these ageless treatments, let's consider the profound simplicity that lies at the root of their effectiveness. What other common instruments might be the key to solving the riddles around the treatment of ankylosing spondylitis?

The gradual rise and fall of heat and cold treatments is evidence of the significant influence of minimalism in the treatment of Ankylosing Spondylitis. Let's continue our journey toward holistic healing by following the hints of wisdom that come from these traditional methods. Together, we can unravel this maze and create new paths.

Mind-Body Techniques

Introduction to the List:

The mind-body link is a crucial component of holistic healthcare and wellness that should not be disregarded. For those with Ankylosing Spondylitis, mind-body therapies like yoga, tai chi, and guided imagery have the potential to be very effective in reducing pain, increasing range of motion, and fostering a state of calm and relaxation. By adopting these practises, you can gain the ability to manage your health and find peace even in the face of the difficulties this illness presents.

Presentation of the List:

1. Yoga: A Path to Alignment and Comfort
2. Tai Chi: Harmonizing Body and Mind
3. Guided Imagery: Harnessing the Power of Visualization

Point Elaboration:

Yoga: A Path to Alignment and Comfort

Yoga is an age-old discipline that integrates the mind, body, and spirit and provides a comprehensive approach to health. Its forceful yet soft postures, along with mindfulness and concentrated breathing, can be especially helpful for people who have ankylosing spondylitis. Yoga strives to create a sense of balance and harmony inside the body by enhancing flexibility, reducing inflammation, and relieving pain through a sequence of carefully planned movements and poses.

Detail Expansion:

Yoga places a strong emphasis on alignment, which is particularly advantageous for people who have ankylosing spondylitis. Yoga maintains and enhances spinal flexibility by gently stretching and strengthening the muscles and ligaments, which stops stiffness from getting worse and encourages a wider range of motion. Moreover, the contemplative nature of yoga fosters an elevated consciousness of the body, empowering people to comprehend and address their physical constraints and requirements more effectively.

Evidence and Testimonials:

Yoga has been shown in numerous studies to have a positive effect on pain management and functional abilities in people with Ankylosing Spondylitis. Additionally, after adding yoga to their daily routine, many people with this illness have experienced considerable increases in overall well-being as well as reductions in pain and stiffness.

Practical Applications:

Including yoga in your routine for self-care can have a profound effect. The gentle movements and attentive breathing of yoga can offer a calming reprieve from the problems of Ankylosing Spondylitis, whether you choose to practise in a class or at home. By practising yoga on a daily basis, you can regain more agency over your body and its health, as well as resilience and empowerment.

Tai Chi: Harmonizing Body and Mind

Tai Chi is an elegant form of exercise with ancient Chinese roots. It is sometimes referred to as "meditation in action." This soft, flowing technique offers a special way to enhance both physical and mental well-being. It blends deliberate, slow movements with concentrated breathing and mental focus. Tai chi offers a chance for people with Ankylosing Spondylitis to develop balance, enhance posture, and lessen pain and stress.

Detail Expansion:

Tai chi's flowing, circular motions are meant to improve the body's natural flow of vital energy, or "qi." People who perform these mild movements can reduce stress in their muscles, improve flexibility in their joints, and cultivate a more relaxed state of mind. Tai chi's meditative qualities also promote mindfulness and help people stay grounded in the present moment by raising awareness of the body and its motions.

Evidence and Testimonials:

Studies on the effects of tai chi on people with ankylosing spondylitis have shown improvements in pain, range of motion, and general quality of life. In addition, a great deal of people have talked about how practising tai chi on a regular basis has helped them personally deal with stiffness and discomfort, highlighting the significant positive effects it has had on both their physical and mental health.

Practical Applications:

Including tai chi in your daily practise can be a gentle yet effective way to deal with the difficulties associated with having ankylosing spondylitis. The methodical, flowing motions of tai chi, whether practised in a group or alone, provide a way to develop both physical and mental fortitude. Adopting tai chi as a regular practise fosters peace and tranquilly, enabling you to face the challenges of this disease head-on with bravery and grace.

Guided Imagery: Harnessing the Power of Visualization

The practise of guided imagery, which entails the use of mental images and visualisation, has the capacity to significantly affect a person's emotional and physical health. People can immerse themselves in vivid, sensory experiences that induce emotions of relaxation, comfort, and healing by using their imagination. Guided imagery is a mild yet effective way to reduce pain, tension, and promote inner peace for those with Ankylosing Spondylitis.

Detail Expansion:

With guided imagery, people are able to generate and interact with mental images that elicit a deep sensation of peace and well-being. People can effectively offset the effects of pain and tension by immersing themselves in scenes of comfort and calm, which induces a state of relaxation that permeates the entire body. People can transcend the limitations of physical suffering and achieve a profound sense of inner calm and contentment by harnessing the power of vision.

Evidence and Testimonials:

Research has shown that guided imagery is effective in lowering stress, anxiety, and discomfort in those with long-term illnesses, such as ankylosing spondylitis. Many people have talked about how they personally found comfort and relief from their conditions by using guided imagery, claiming the technique's capacity to offer a therapeutic haven in the middle of their illness's difficulties.

Practical Applications:

Including guided imagery in your daily practise can be a game-changer when it comes to controlling the effects of ankylosing spondylitis on your health. The practise of guided imaging provides a haven of peace and comfort, whether through customised visualisation exercises or guided meditation recordings. This allows people to manage the intricacies of their disease with resilience and serenity. By making guided visualisation a daily practise, you can go beyond the limits of physical suffering and achieve a profound sense of inner calm and well-being.

Seamless Transitions:

A game-changer for controlling the effects of Ankylosing Spondylitis on your health is to include guided imagery into your everyday routine. Through the use of customised visualisation exercises or guided meditation recordings, guided imagery provides a peaceful and comforting haven that helps people deal with the intricacies of their disease in a resilient and peaceful manner. You can achieve a deep sense of inner calm and wellbeing by regularly using guided imagery, which goes beyond the realm of physical discomfort.

Supportive Therapies

: Nurturing the Body and Soul

Upon delving into the complex maze of managing Ankylosing Spondylitis, it is evident that our path extends beyond the domain of physical well-being. This ailment presents equally major emotional and practical obstacles, necessitating a comprehensive strategy that goes beyond traditional therapeutic approaches. This subchapter explores the powerful effects of supportive therapies, such as occupational therapy, counselling, and support groups, on body and soul nourishment, resilience building, and enabling people to survive in the face of the severe obstacles presented by ankylosing spondylitis.

Imagine a calm, sunlit space that is decorated with vivid colours and the soft glow of natural light. People congregate here in the calm of this area, creating a patchwork of mutual experiences and tacit understanding. Everybody has their own weight to bear, but in this sanctuary, the promise of healing and the warmth of compassion provide comfort.

Introducing Sarah, a vibrant young lady whose life was permanently changed when she developed Ankylosing Spondylitis. The constant pain that pierced her entire existence threw a shadow over her hopes and desires, overshadowing her formerly joyful attitude. However, she found a loving environment and a group of committed experts within these walls who worked to restore not only her physical health but also her joy and sense of purpose.

One component of ankylosing spondylitis that is frequently disregarded is the emotional toll it takes. The lives of those impacted may be permeated with feelings of melancholy, worry, and isolation, making the already difficult process of treating the physical symptoms much more difficult. In addition, real-world difficulties like adjusting to a new lifestyle and figuring out the intricacies of everyday chores can be quite difficult.

Counseling seems as a ray of hope, providing a platform for people to express their deepest worries and thoughts as well as to work through the range of emotions that come with the trip. Individuals can learn to reframe their thoughts, build resilience, and create coping techniques that act as pillars of strength in the face of adversity through customised therapies.

Support groups also act as a mosaic of common experiences, where members are surrounded by a tapestry of compassion and understanding. Here, amidst their loneliness, individuals discover camaraderie and gain insight from the combined successes and setbacks of their peers.

Occupational therapy plays a crucial role in providing people with the skills and strategies they need to deal with the day-to-day obstacles of life. Occupational therapists help people regain their independence and autonomy by providing ergonomic solutions and adaptive methods. This helps people feel like they have agency outside the constraints of their condition.

These supportive therapies have a tangible transforming effect. Sarah used to be entangled by the entanglement of hopelessness, but she now exudes a fresh sense of life and purpose. Her involvement in therapy has given her a strong sense of self-awareness and emotional fortitude, which empowers her to face the challenges of Ankylosing Spondylitis head-on. Her haven is now the support group, which gives her days a spirit-encouraging sense of understanding and togetherness. She has regained a sense of agency in her day-to-day activities because to the practical tactics and adaptive techniques she has learned via occupational therapy.

Sarah's storey highlights the critical role supportive therapies play in promoting overall wellbeing. It also makes us consider how often the psychological and practical difficulties caused by ankylosing spondylitis are underestimated. It is critical that we acknowledge the fundamental connections between mental and physical health and give supportive therapy top priority when incorporating it into all-encompassing treatment plans.

This subchapter is accompanied by powerful pictures that encapsulate the core of these supportive therapies—a visual representation of the transformative power of empathy, comprehension, and empowerment.

Sarah's storey goes beyond the parameters of her personal experience and speaks to the experiences of many who are attempting to make their way through the maze of Ankylosing Spondylitis. It emphasises how supportive therapies may change people's lives by building resilience, developing empathy, and rekindling hope in their hearts.

Let us consider the great importance of mental health in the context of Ankylosing Spondylitis as we begin this investigation into supportive therapy. In what ways might incorporating supportive therapies into our management techniques lead to a more humane and comprehensive approach to healthcare? In the pages that follow, join us as we unravel the healing and empowering tangle.

Creating a Personalized Ankylosing Spondylitis Management Plan

Assessing Your Symptoms and Needs

Greetings from the gateway to self-discovery and empowerment on your path to conquering Ankylosing Spondylitis, dear reader. We take a comprehensive look at your particular symptoms, needs, and goals in this subchapter, setting the foundation for a personalised Ankylosing Spondylitis treatment plan that speaks to your own spirit.

Our goal is to lead you on a contemplative journey that reveals the nuances of your Ankylosing Spondylitis experience and produces a customised treatment plan for all-encompassing care.

All you need is an open heart, the desire to explore the depths of your being, and a quiet place where you can spend time connecting with your deepest self to begin this introspective trip.

First, we will softly highlight the terrain of your demands and symptoms, illuminating the subtleties that mould your day-to-day life. After that, we will navigate the maze of self-awareness and reveal the interwoven strands of your mental, emotional, and spiritual health.

Allow me to invite you to open your senses to the whispers of your body, mind, and soul as we embark on this holy excursion. Spend a moment writing in your notebook about your experiences, carefully noting the rise and fall of your symptoms. While you're at it, let your mind wander through your heart's hallways to reveal the emotional fabric that's woven throughout your physical journey.

After that, we'll start a cautious investigation into your everyday requirements, piecing together a nuanced portrait of your relationships, way of life, and goals. Talk to yourself thoughtfully, recognising the aspects of your life that support and nurture you in addition to those that require gentle attention and change.

Be kind to yourself as you navigate this delicate terrain, reader. Accept the whole range of your experiences with grace and compassion. Let the pen glide across the pages of your diary, creating a mosaic of your deepest emotions and ideas. Recall that the true melody of your being is the only thing that matters, not right or wrong replies.

It's OK to feel things in this gentle question that might make your soul sing. Honor the holiness of your path by tenderly embracing these moments. In the event that you become overwhelmed, gently bring your attention to the calming pattern of your breathing and ground yourself in the here and now.

After sifting through the maze of your demands and symptoms, stop briefly to admire the mosaic of realisations that have appeared. Let your eyes rest on the details of your encounter, following the curves of your path with awe.

Once you've given some thought to your journal entries and the gentle self-talk you've established, carefully condense the substance of your experience down to a few essential observations. These priceless discoveries will form the cornerstone of your customised Ankylosing Spondylitis treatment strategy, providing direction and clarity for your future steps.

This sensitive examination, my reader, is evidence of your bravery and tenacity. You are embracing the entirety of your being with grace and compassion as you weave the tapestry of your own recovery path with every step.

I encourage you to treat yourself with tolerance and love if you encounter resistance or uncertainty while on this introspective trip. Accept the uncomfortable times as mild invitations to explore your inner wisdom more deeply. Know that you are not alone if you need advice or assistance. Seek out empathetic individuals who are willing to join you on this holy journey of self-exploration.

May you take the soft murmurs of your heart with you as we pull back the curtain on this intimate inquiry. Accept the bright fabric of your existence with reverence, for it contains the design for your individual Ankylosing Spondylitis treatment strategy.

Breathe in the essence of your journey in the quiet of this vulnerable moment. Recognize that you are deserving of the boundless grace that awaits you and that you are in control of your own healing.

With light and love,
Dr. Ankita Kashyap

Setting Realistic Goals

Greetings and welcome to a life-changing adventure as you learn to effectively manage your Ankylosing Spondylitis. Setting reasonable and attainable goals will be crucial to our success as we travel this route together. We will discuss the importance of goal-setting in this subchapter, as well as the possible repercussions of skipping this important phase. We will also offer doable, research-backed strategies to help you on your path to recovery.

Let's set the stage by discussing the significant influence goal-setting can have on controlling ankylosing spondylitis before we get into the specifics of goal-setting. When it comes to holistic health and wellbeing, establishing meaningful goals is like laying out a road map for a better, healthier future. It acts as a compass, pointing people in the direction of a resilient, balanced existence.

The main problem at hand is the propensity to undervalue the significance of realistic goal-setting in the treatment of ankylosing spondylitis. Without specific goals and objectives, people could find themselves lost in an ocean of doubt and unable to fully utilise their healing process.

Ignoring the important work of goal-setting might have serious repercussions. People may feel aimless in the absence of a clear goal, which can cause them to become frustrated, feel powerless, and lose motivation to pursue the essential lifestyle changes and self-care routines. This may lead to a halt in advancement and a decline in standard of living.

We suggest a strategy based on empowerment and individualised treatment to meet this difficulty. We may create the conditions for long-term development and comprehensive well-being by establishing reasonable and doable goals that are suited to each person's preferences, talents, and lifestyle. By putting the person at the centre of their own recovery process, this method promotes empowerment and a sense of ownership.

The first step in putting this idea into practise is to gain a thorough grasp of each person's particular situation, goals, and difficulties. We are able to create a meaningful and achievable road map by working together with wellness specialists, healthcare providers, and the individual. This could entail dividing big objectives into smaller, achievable milestones and combining food changes, self-care routines, lifestyle alterations, and coping mechanisms.

The effectiveness of this strategy is demonstrated by the significant changes that people who have embraced the power of setting realistic goals have undergone. People have reported increased motivation, a fresh sense of purpose, and noticeable gains in their mental and physical health when their goals are in line with their ability. The aforementioned data substantiates the revolutionary potential of customised goal-setting in the treatment of Ankylosing Spondylitis.

Even though the suggested approach has a lot of potential, it's important to recognise that there might be other options. But the beauty of customised goal-setting is that it respects each person's own path, encouraging autonomy and self-determination. This method embraces the complex nature of healing and wellbeing, going beyond one-size-fits-all fixes.

Let's add some charm and whimsy to this process as we go through the nuances of creating achievable goals. Imagine the delicately unfurling petals of a flower; each one signifies a step closer to your goals. Accept the gentle, visceral picture of a calm garden, where every objective is a seed that is intentionally planted and grown.

In the pages that follow, we will delve into the subtleties of customising these aspirations to meet specific requirements and tastes as we examine the artistry of creating objectives that are both meaningful and attainable. One objective at a time, together, we shall illuminate the way towards holistic well-being.

So let's begin this enchanted adventure of goal-setting, dear reader, armed with the knowledge of individualised care and the transformational force of self-empowerment. Your unique goal-setting blueprint, filled with resilience, hope, and gentle direction, is waiting for you. It is the blueprint for managing Ankylosing Spondylitis completely.

Building a Support Network

Here we are, reader, at the centre of the trip with Ankylosing Spondylitis. We are forced to face the indisputable fact that no one can traverse this route alone as we delve deeper into the complex web of treating this disease. Because of its mysterious character, ankylosing spondylitis necessitates a multimodal approach to management, and the foundation of this strategy is the important support network.

Ankylosing Spondylitis is a chronic inflammatory arthritis that mostly affects the spine. It can damage a person's physical, emotional, and mental health, among other areas of their life. A comprehensive approach to care and management is necessary because the difficulties this condition presents frequently transcend the boundaries of traditional medical care.

The main problem is the sense of loneliness that can overcome people who are attempting to navigate the maze of Ankylosing Spondylitis. In the absence of a strong support system, the burden of chronic illness can become too much to bear, leaving one feeling hopeless and hopeless.

The ramifications of managing Ankylosing Spondylitis in isolation can be severe. The lack of a supporting community can make this condition more difficult to manage, resulting in symptoms including anxiety and feelings of isolation as well as difficulties adhering to treatment regimens.

Building a support system is where the light of hope rests on this journey. This network is a constellation of people and resources, not just a safety net, that can light the way ahead and give you the courage and fortitude to tackle the challenges posed by ankylosing spondylitis.

Creating a support system requires a diversified strategy. The foundation of this network is, first and foremost, drawing on the knowledge of medical specialists, such as rheumatologists, physical therapists, and mental health specialists. The embrace of friends, family, and support groups can also offer priceless practical and emotional help. Incorporating alternative therapies and self-care routines can strengthen this network even further and provide new channels of support.

It is often known that having a strong support system helps manage chronic diseases. Research has demonstrated that people with robust support systems enjoy greater overall quality of life, better treatment adherence, and higher emotional well-being. People with Ankylosing Spondylitis can experience a more resilient and powerful journey by fostering this network and utilising the combined strength and wisdom of their group.

While each person's journey towards creating a support system will be unique, some other options include using online forums to get peer support, practising mindfulness and relaxation techniques, and finding creative outlets like music therapy and art. These other options can enhance the management of ankylosing spondylitis overall by acting as complimentary strands in the complex web of a support system.

As we go out on this journey to create a support system, picture a tapestry woven with the brilliant colours of knowledge, compassion, and understanding. From the unfailing warmth of loved ones to the delicate counsel of healthcare professionals, each thread symbolises an essential element of this network. These strands come together to form a strong fabric that supports and comforts people navigating the maze that is ankylosing spondylitis.

We will go deeper into the skill of creating this support system, examine the subtleties of incorporating medical knowledge, cultivate emotional forbearance, and embrace the transforming potential of holistic wellness in the upcoming chapters. Let's go out on this journey with open minds and hearts as the embrace of a caring support system holds the key to resilience and empowerment in the face of ankylosing spondylitis.

As we bid each other farewell for the time being, picture the breaking of a new dawn where the chorus of support resounds with unflinching compassion and strength. May the seeds of your support system grow and bloom, providing comfort and strength on your Ankylosing Spondylitis journey, till we cross paths again, dear reader.

Developing Self-Care Techniques

Introduction to the List:

With Ankylosing Spondylitis, self-care becomes an essential tool in our toolbox as we learn to manage its complexities. By taking care of our mental, emotional, and physical health, we may reduce the symptoms of our illness and develop a healthy relationship with our bodies. We will examine a carefully chosen range of self-care methods in this subchapter, all aimed at empowering you to achieve holistic wellness.

Presentation of the List:

1. Stress Management
2. Relaxation Exercises
3. Lifestyle Modifications

Point Elaboration:

Stress Management

Breathing Methods for Reducing Stress

b. When stress levels are at an all-time high, our breath acts as a lifeline, bringing us back to the present and settling the turbulent waves inside. Deliberate breathing techniques, such diaphragmatic or box breathing, help us relax our nerve systems and lessen the negative effects of stress on our bodies.

c. Studies have demonstrated that deep breathing exercises can considerably lower felt tension and anxiety, providing a concrete route toward emotional balance.

d. Real-World Uses: Include these breathing techniques in your everyday practise, particularly for times when you're feeling upset or uncomfortable. Through the practise of aware breathing, you may bring peace and balance into your day.

Relaxation Exercises

A Guided Relaxation Imagery

b. Allow me to take you on a peaceful journey within our thoughts. Guided imagery, sometimes referred to as visualisation, takes us to quiet settings and surrounds us with peace, promoting deep relaxation and mental renewal.

c. Studies on clinical trials have shown how effective guided imagery is at lowering pain and fostering relaxation; this makes it a non-invasive option for treating Ankylosing Spondylitis-related discomfort.

d. Real-World Uses: Allocate a specific time for guided imagery sessions, and give yourself permission to lose yourself in the calming scenes your mind creates. By incorporating this technique into your daily routine, you can use visualization's healing properties to release stress in both your body and mind.

Lifestyle Modifications

a. Ergonomic Workstation Setup

b. The way our workstations are designed has a significant impact on our overall well-being as does our physical surroundings. We may reduce the pressure on our bodies, promote comfort, and lessen the influence of Ankylosing Spondylitis on our everyday activities by maximising our workspace using ergonomic concepts.

c. The testimonials of those who have made ergonomic adjustments to their workstations highlight the revolutionary effect of this transformation, attesting to the reduction of discomfort and the recovery of productivity.

d. Useful Applications: Assess your workspace and make ergonomic changes, including adding lumbar support or modifying the height of your desk and chair. By designing your office with your body in mind, you may strengthen your resistance to the difficulties that Ankylosing Spondylitis presents.

Seamless Transitions:

Every thread in the self-care tapestry adds something special to the overall harmony of our wellbeing. We uncover a range of techniques that align the rhythm of our lives with the tune of holistic wellbeing as we explore the nuances of stress management, relaxation techniques, and lifestyle adjustments. As we embrace the transforming power of these self-care approaches, let's continue our exploration.

Adapting to Flare-Ups

We go through the complex terrain of Ankylosing Spondylitis, experiencing highs and lows, periods of fortitude and resiliency, and moments when the unpredictable nature of this illness manifests itself as flare-ups. These don't have to be intimidating; they can be difficult. We'll look at how to adjust to flare-ups in this chapter, and how to ride the ups and downs with grace, fortitude, and a steady attitude.

Imagine this: With Ankylosing Spondylitis, you've been navigating the calm seas of your everyday schedule and discovering your rhythm in the ups and downs of life. Unexpectedly, a flare-up appears out of nowhere, clouding your carefully thought-out plans and habits. It's like a soft wind has turned into a hurricane, upsetting the peace you've worked so hard to create.

Ankylosing spondylitis flare-ups can cause episodes of increased pain, stiffness, and exhaustion, upsetting the delicate equilibrium you've worked so hard to establish. These abrupt increases can have an adverse effect on your emotional and mental fortitude in addition to your physical health.

Flickers that go untreated can make you feel frustrated and powerless, which can make it harder for you to go about your daily business, work, and interact with people. These flare-ups can have a knock-on effect that penetrates your emotional and mental health in addition to the physical world.

When faced with a flare-up, there is a wealth of coping tactics and techniques to help you get through it. Through the adoption of a comprehensive strategy that addresses mental and physical health, we can create a manual for resiliency and strength in the face of flare-ups.

1. A customised pain management strategy, ranging from heat therapy and mindfulness exercises to mild stretches and targeted activities, can offer relief during flare-ups.

2. You can manage flare-ups more easily by implementing little changes to your daily schedule, such pacing yourself, organising your workspace, and scheduling restorative breaks.

3. Building a supportive community, taking part in stress-relieving activities, and adopting an optimistic outlook can strengthen your emotional resilience when experiencing emotional outbursts.

In spite of the unpredictable nature of ankylosing spondylitis, you can develop a sense of agency and empowerment by including these tactics into your flare-up management toolkit. Patients have reported improvements in overall quality of life due to decreased intensity and length of flare-ups, customised pain management, and adjustments to everyday activities that foster emotional resilience.

Although the aforementioned tactics provide a strong basis for managing flare-ups, it's important to understand that every person's experience with Ankylosing Spondylitis is different. Examining complementary therapies like hydrotherapy, biofeedback, or acupuncture in addition to traditional methods can provide a multimodal strategy to controlling flare-ups.

Remind yourself that you are not alone as you go out on this journey of learning to live with flare-ups. When we band together, we can weather the storms with resolute fortitude and a spirit that won't be crushed by doubt's gloom.

We will go further into the nuances of pain management, the skill of adjusting everyday activities, and the gentle development of mental resilience in the upcoming chapters, creating a comprehensive plan for managing Ankylosing Spondylitis from head to toe. Together, let's set out on this life-changing adventure, negotiating the highs and lows with discernment, grace, and an unwavering spirit.

Monitoring and Tracking Progress

Greetings from the chapter that is the core of your path to becoming an expert in managing your Ankylosing Spondylitis. We will discuss the critical skill of recording and monitoring your progress in these pages, which is an important step toward full treatment of your Ankylosing Spondylitis. As you take daily responsibility for your health and well-being, it is imperative that you remain vigilant about how your symptoms, medications, and lifestyle choices change over time. Together, let's go on this insightful journey to discover the game-changing potential of tracking and monitoring.

Your goal is apparent: to become well-versed in how your body reacts to different treatments and to proactively pursue optimal wellness. You will be able to create management plans that are specifically suited to your needs by keeping an eye on your progress and tracking it in order to spot trends, turning points, and accomplishments.

A few basic tools will help you accomplish this goal: a symptom diary specifically for recording symptoms, a way to monitor the efficacy of medications, and a way to assess lifestyle modifications. Throughout this journey, these tools will be your devoted friends, helping you to gain vital insights into the rhythms and responses of your body.

A key component of tracking and monitoring progress is the delicate skill of observation. It takes acute awareness and a caring relationship with your body and mind to get through this process. You will acquire a greater comprehension of the complex dance between your decisions and their effects on your well-being via a series of attentive practises. In order to cultivate a harmonious balance within, we will investigate the rhythm of your symptoms, the ups and downs of pharmaceutical efficacy, and the minute changes in your lifestyle choices.

1. Start by making a straightforward yet thorough symptom diary. Your daily experiences will be preserved in this diary, which will also capture the subtleties of your mental and physical health. Note how

much pain you are experiencing, how well you are sleeping, whether you are tired or stiff, and whether your emotions are changing. You will eventually identify trends and triggers by keeping track of these specifics, which will empower you to make well-informed decisions regarding your way of life and course of therapy.

2. It's crucial to monitor the efficacy of your drugs concurrently. Keep track of the dates on which you take your doses, the comfort they bring, and any possible adverse effects. Your treatment plan will be optimised by individualised adjustments that result from this close monitoring, which will enable you to conduct knowledgeable conversations with your healthcare team.

3. It's important to assess the effects of any lifestyle changes you make, including eating adjustments, stress reduction methods, and exercise regimens. Maintain a journal of your activities and the results you get so you may identify the practises that are most in tune with your body and soul.

- Accept the tracking and monitoring procedure with an attitude of self-compassion and mild curiosity. Refrain from passing judgement or criticising yourself because of what you have noticed. Rather, see each realisation as a priceless jewel that points you in the direction of increased wellbeing.

- Recall that development could happen in discrete, complex ways. It's possible that even seemingly insignificant changes to your everyday routine can have far-reaching effects.

Validate that this practise was completed successfully by thinking back on your capacity to identify trends and triggers, having educated conversations with your healthcare team, and acting with confidence after reviewing your findings. Your commitment to holistic wellness is demonstrated by this continuous journey of self-discovery and improvement.

Rely on the assistance of your medical team and the experience of other people who have travelled this route in case you encounter difficulties or uncertainties. Seek advice, pose inquiries, and have an open mind to fresh viewpoints that can help you on your path.

Let these activities' soft rhythms become a calming song in the wellness journey as you immerse yourself in the skill of measuring and monitoring progress. With a heart full of optimism and a spirit tuned in to your body's whispers, embrace every observation, every insight, and every stride forward. We will delve into the transforming potential of self-care strategies in the upcoming chapter, while you continue to tend to a deep wellspring of inner resilience. Until then, may you be led by the subtle art of tracking and monitoring to a life full of vitality and harmony.

Adjusting the Management Plan

We have to accept that our route is not always clear-cut when we set out to learn the nuances of controlling ankylosing spondylitis. Our health and well-being fluctuate in the same way as the natural world does. It's okay if the management plan we create today needs to be adjusted tomorrow. It's actually perfectly fine—a it's normal component of the procedure. Let's now explore the skill of modifying our management plan to keep it as flexible and adaptable as we are.

Imagine yourself as someone who has been faithfully adhering to your management plan, enjoying the soothing rhythms of self-care practises, fueling your body with healthful foods, and appreciating the assistance of your healthcare team. But something doesn't feel right. It's possible that your symptoms are changing or that your lifestyle has changed. Our management plan has to adapt to these times of change in order to suit our needs now.

The main difficulty we have is keeping our management plan up to date with the constantly shifting circumstances in our lives. Ankylosing Spondylitis is a disease that moves to the rhythm of our individual experiences rather than following a set of rigid guidelines. This means that our management strategy needs to be adaptable and flexible enough to change as our situation does.

We run the risk of feeling out of step with our body and the changing course of our illness if we fail to make the necessary adjustments to our management strategy. Increased discomfort, a feeling of helplessness, and a misalignment with our general well-being could result from this connection. We run the danger of passing up chances to enhance our quality of life and more effectively manage our symptoms if we ignore the need for modifications.

Embracing the skill of adaptability is the answer. We have to develop an attitude that is open to change, realising that our management plan is a live, breathing document that will change and grow with us. This entails keeping an open mind, looking for novel methods, and incorporating brand-new information into our strategy.

Self-awareness and proactive participation are the cornerstones of the steps involved in incorporating improvements into our management strategy. Start by becoming aware of your body's signals and recording any changes in general wellbeing or symptom shifts. Engage in open communication with your healthcare staff, offering insights and working together to identify possible improvements. Seize the chance to experiment with new self-care methods, dietary changes, and lifestyle choices that suit your current situation.

We can achieve better symptom management, a higher quality of life, and a stronger sense of empowerment by accepting the flexibility of our treatment plan. Previous experiences have demonstrated that individuals who modify their treatment plan to accommodate their changing needs frequently have a more positive relationship with their illness, which promotes resilience and a higher sense of well-being.

Although being flexible is crucial, it's important to think about additional options that might work in addition to our main plan. These can be looking into complementary therapies, getting more advice from health professionals, or incorporating mindfulness exercises into our regular routines. All these paths have the capacity to enhance our management strategy and promote our general welfare.

Let us approach the process of fine-tuning our management strategy with an open mind and a curious attitude. Think of it like a slow dance, where we flow through life, integrating new steps and moves with elegance as we sway in time with our evolving demands. Accepting the flexibility of our management plan is a call to take a closer look at our wellbeing and to acknowledge that it is a gracefully winding path that we walk with fortitude and grace rather than a straight line. This is the key to managing ankylosing spondylitis: navigating its complexities with compassion and flexibility rather than blindly following a prescribed course.